Sleep Secrets: Switch off your brain, sleep better, and feel refreshed in just 9 easy steps

And so it begins

It's 2am on a Monday morning. You're still awake. Wide awake. Staring at the ceiling yet again, worrying every 10 minutes about how much time you have left to sleep before you have to get up for work. The more you try to close your eyes and concentrate on falling asleep, the harder it seems to be. It's a vicious cycle. You're exhausted and frustrated, but your brain just won't 'click' off.

I've been there: for six months I relied on the little sleep I got to keep functioning. If I managed four hours, it was a great night, but when it started dropping to two hours, then one hour, then 20 minutes, I knew I had to do something! Anything! I was in a state of turmoil, and it seemed as though nothing was helping, which simply made my frustration worse. It started affecting my mood, my work and my relationships. I had to find a way. It took months trying to figure out what it was that was keeping me awake. I was willing to try anything out of sheer desperation.

Then one day I got it right.

Is this the book for you?

If, like me, you are at that point where you are feeling frustrated and you just need to sleep, then this book is for you. I have taken the time to meticulously compile everything I've tried into one small, easy-to-follow guide in the hopes that my experiences could somehow help you. I've also included short action plans for each step to really give you a head start. You will learn how to give yourself every advantage to fall asleep, from getting your environment ready to monitoring your patterns with a sleep log and trying various techniques on how to relax a busy mind.

The purpose of this book is purely to help you figure out what is keeping you awake and how we can possibly fix that together.

So if you're ready for some serious shut-eye, then let's get started!

Contents

Step 7: The ultimate chill-out guide

First, the facts

If you're reading this book, then I'm sure you know what insomnia is, but just to put it into words, there are two main types of insomnia. Firstly, there is the inability to fall asleep, and secondly, the inability to stay asleep long enough to function like a normal human being the next day. Your brain releases two separate hormones to help you fall asleep and stay asleep, but various contributing factors can inhibit them. When this happens, as with my own experience, your body is naturally physically tired, but your brain won't switch off at all because it won't release the chemicals needed for a decent sleep cycle.

If you have suffered from any of the below for an extended period of time, you might have insomnia.

- You can't fall asleep.
- You can't stay asleep or get back to sleep.
- You wake up all the time during the night.
- You wake up too early in the morning.
- You feel tired and drowsy the next day.
- You start noticing changes in your mood.
- You rely on sleeping tablets or alcohol to fall asleep.

Insomnia is also very much a conditioned or learned action. You progressively tend to get worse, or it gets harder to fall asleep as you start to become anxious and stressed about the fact that you are not sleeping. This shows it is imperative to re-create and establish a relaxed sleeping environment and mindset in order to stop this vicious cycle.

What needs to be clearly noted early on in this book is that everyone's insomnia is made up of a different cocktail of smaller underlying issues. What may work for one person will not necessarily work for the next. This is why I've tried to develop this easy-to-follow, holistic guide, with not only tips and tricks that helped me to get over my six-month insomnia, but also other options that may help you as well. It tends to take some time to figure out what your underlying issues are, so be patient with yourself and do your best to monitor your progress over a reasonable amount of time. I worked with two weeks, slowly adding more techniques to my sleep regimen. You may find you need a little more time or even less depending on the severity of your insomnia.

What causes insomnia?

There are many different causes for insomnia, the most common of which are anxiety, stress and diet. You could be suffering from physical, mental or medical issues that are inhibiting your sleep patterns.

Physical issues can be boiled down to the type of sleeping environment you have, the lifestyle you lead, which includes alcohol and drug use, as well as daytime habits.

Mental issues would include stress, anxiety and depression or other mental illnesses. Mental issues tend to be the root cause of half of insomnia cases, and take a lot longer to treat. Natural treatments are not a guarantee for curing these kinds of insomnia, but are very often an easy method of providing relief.

There are also medical issues that may be causing your insomnia. This could be anything from asthma and acid reflux to chronic pain and kidney problems. If you suspect you have a medical problem, you should consult your GP. The strange thing about insomnia is that it could also just be a side effect of a completely separate sleep disorder you are suffering from, such as restless leg syndrome or sleep apnoea. Restless leg syndrome is a tingling or painful feeling in your leg that keeps you awake, and sleep apnoea is a break in your natural breathing pattern that causes you to wake up through the night.

What if I don't get enough sleep?

When there is a lack of sleep, your brain is unable to recharge properly, and this makes it difficult not only to concentrate and take in new information or learn new things, but it could even lead to poor decision making and problem solving. You could find it difficult to control your emotions and behaviour, and may even become depressed or prone to mood swings over time. In a work environment your judgement may be impaired and your reaction time can slow. One could easily see how this could jeopardise your relationships and career if prolonged over time.

Because sleep is directly involved in repairing your physical body, it is safe to then assume that a lack of sleep could lead to bodily complications, such as heart disease, high blood pressure, and even a depleted immune system. It can also result in weight gain as sleep affects the hormone responsible for making us feel hungry.

Even a small lack of sleep over a few days could lead to something called 'microsleep'. This is where you basically fall asleep for tiny periods of time when you're actually awake. As complicated as that may sound it is really quite simple to explain. Have you ever driven somewhere and when you finally reach your destination you can't quite completely remember driving the whole way? You could have experienced microsleep. Studies show that a sleep deficiency is possibly even more dangerous than alcohol behind the wheel of a car. This is a small example of how a lack of sleep could affect your life, or the life of another for that matter.

How much shut-eye do I really need?

Different strokes for different folks. Some people need seven hours, and some need eight to nine hours of sleep, which is considered to be the norm. This is very often based on your age and how strenuous your daily activities are. Normal sleep essentially means falling asleep easily when going to bed (after up to 15 minutes) and thereafter experiencing the four stages of the sleep cycle. These stages are as follows:

Stage 1 is the lightest stage of sleep. Your eyes are closed at this point but you are still easily awakened, feeling as though you probably haven't slept yet.
Stage 2 is the stage where people spend most of their sleep. This is where your mind relaxes and focuses more on rest and 'turning off', and becomes somehow unaware of what's happening around you. Your heart rate will slow and your bodily temperature will cool down.
Stage 3 is even deeper and is the stage at which your body starts to heal itself.
Stage 4 is where rapid eye movement (REM) sleep happens. This is said to be the stage in which you have the most vivid dreams, and where your mind is most active. You could also experience a 'paralysed' effect in this stage.

Step 1: Get prepared and get positive

1.1 The insomniac's checklist

I've created the below checklist purely as a base point to help you try to figure out what is causing your insomnia. I suggest you tick or write down what applies to you, and keep this in mind when writing in your sleep diary, which we will chat about in 1.2.

General issues	Yes/No
Do you struggle to fall asleep?	
Do you struggle to stay asleep?	
Are you becoming frustrated with not being able to fall asleep?	
Are you currently menstruating, experiencing menopause or pregnant?	
Do you struggle to fall asleep?	
Do you struggle to stay asleep?	
Are you becoming frustrated with not being able to fall asleep?	
Examples likely to be a physical issue:	**Yes/No**
Did your environment or location change recently?	
Did your lifestyle change recently?	
Are you naturally a light sleeper?	
Is your bedroom bright?	
Is your bedroom noisy?	
Are your bed and pillow uncomfortable?	
Do you use LED-lit devices late into the night or in bed?	
Do you struggle to exercise on a regular basis?	
Do you exercise in the morning or evening?	
Have you flown for long periods of time	

recently?	
Has your work shift changed recently?	
Has your diet changed recently?	
Examples likely to be a mental issue:	**Yes/No**
Do you find you lie awake worrying about things when you go to bed?	
Are you stressing about things at work?	
Do you argue with your partner or spouse in the bedroom?	
Do you work on your laptop in the bedroom?	
Does anyone in your family suffer from insomnia?	
Do you feel depressed, anxious or worried?	
Do you find you lie awake worrying about things when you go to bed?	
Are you stressing about things at work?	

While going through these steps you may find that not just one technique works, but a number of separate techniques all together.

1.2 A super-simple sleep log

In order to start this nine-step guide to better sleep, I want you to get a book and a pen and label this your "sleep diary". While going through these steps over the next few weeks, I want you to write down in short descriptions what your activity is like in the day and how well you sleep at night (or not at all in this case).

By monitoring what activities you do before going to bed, what time you go to bed and how long it actually took you to fall asleep, you'll be able to easily pick up on patterns affecting your sleep.

I've put together a short list of questions I answered about my day when I got home to try and establish my pattern. I suggest using mine as a base of reference and to simply add and adapt it to your own lifestyle to better monitor your own sleeping habits.

My sleep log:

Day 1	
Action	Answer
What time did I wake up this morning?	
How did I feel when I woke up? Was I stiff, uncomfortable or tired?	
How much caffeine did I have during the day?	
What did I eat for breakfast? It's the most important meal of the day!	
What did I eat for lunch?	
What did I eat for supper?	
Did I snack on items containing sugar in the afternoon or at night?	
What time did I go to bed?	
Roughly what time do I think I fell asleep?	
How often did I wake up last night?	
Was there something in my surroundings that woke me up?	
Was there something I was worrying about before falling asleep?	

1.3 Turn that frown upside down

It is important to note that as with any programme, positivity and determination play a large part in your personal success. A great suggestion I once read that helped me start my journey was to repeat positive phrases before going to bed to make sure I slowly stopped associating sleep as such an anxious and daunting task. I would follow the sleep ritual I developed, and as I lay in bed I would repeat to myself:

"One day I will fall asleep with ease. It will be relaxing and peaceful."
"While it may not happen right away, it is not life-threatening."
"I am positive and motivated enough to give myself the best possible chance at falling asleep naturally."

By repeating this softly a few times to myself, sleep became less of a matter of anxiety and performance, and more a mere matter of time.

Action plan 1

1. Go through the insomniac's checklist and on the first page write down what possible causes stood out to you the most. You could even highlight the main problems if you can already identify what they are.

2. On the second page write down a list of questions (you could use mine as a reference) you are going to monitor yourself on over the next few days. Try to keep these related to the causes you may have discovered from your checklist.

3. On your next page, write down a few positive affirmations you could use to calm yourself when getting anxious about falling asleep.

Step 2: Welcome to my palace

A great starting point is to change your sleeping environment. Sometimes we get so busy with our lives that everyday actions become second nature, and we may not even realise that they are actually disrupting or could be disrupting our sleep. For example, if you've recently started getting into some kind of social media posting and are constantly on your mobile phone at night, the LED light could be what's stopping the signals to your brain that tell it it's time to turn off.

2.1 Safety first

It's very difficult to fall asleep if you don't feel completely safe in your environment. This is definitely one of the reasons I suffered from anxiety, which then fed my insomnia. We had a house robbery when I was a young girl and it affected me so much I was always sleeping with one eye open. This is one of the trickier issues to deal with, but it would depend on your situation. In my case I felt safer when we got a dog, but in your case it could mean installing an alarm system or simply a flood light in your garden. This is not to say safety would be a cause of everyone's sleepless nights, but it is well worth considering.

2.2 The bat cave

Turn your bedroom into a bat cave. I would suggest getting black-out curtains to block out as much light as possible. You want to expose yourself to a healthy amount of light in the day, such as a well-lit working environment if you work in an office, or do your best to step outside and work in natural light. Then at bedtime don't expose yourself to any light. The lack of light will make the room less distracting for you, and should cause your brain to realise it is bedtime. You can also try using a sleep mask.

2.3 Get comfortable

Get the right mattress. A mattress that is too soft or too hard could easily inhibit your sleep. I didn't even realise that you actually need to take your body type into consideration when buying a mattress. For example, curvy people need a softer mattress to be able to hold their figure properly, as opposed to pushing against their hips and shoulders. People with a much straighter figure actually need a harder mattress for better support. You should also check your mattress twice a year for wear and tear.

On this note, you should also get the right pillow for your sleeping position and to give yourself enough neck support.

I would advise making sure your pyjamas are as comfortable and breathable as possible. Hot or heavy pyjamas make for a restless night, as we will learn a little later on.

2.4 Say no to disco

At least two hours before bed, try to cut your exposure to screen light on your phone, computer or TV. The LED light emitted from devices act as a stimulant and will make it harder for you to fall asleep.

2.5 Turn down for what?

Try wearing earplugs if you're a light sleeper. Many people are worried that they will completely block out any and all noise, but what they actually do is just drone out the slight changes in noise that tend to keep you awake, like the ticking of your alarm clock or the dog barking outside your window. They don't drown out all noise completely, they just give you the freedom to not feel disturbed or distracted by it.

2.6 It's getting hot in here

Many people would agree that trying to fall asleep on a hot night is extremely frustrating. The heat seems to affect not just your body temperature, but also your brain's ability to relax and concentrate on winding down. This may be linked to the fact that cooler temperatures tend to cool your brain down, requiring less metabolic activity. The less active your brain is, the easier it should be to fall asleep. Try to opt for sleeping with a light fan or cool breeze at night as well as light, comfortable clothing.

2.7 Tick-tock stop the clock

Remove any clocks in your room, and after setting your alarm, put your phone or alarm out of sight or out of arm's reach. Not only does this help with the horrid repetitive ticking, but I've found this also helps with relieving anxiety attached to falling asleep, as you cannot constantly see how much time you have left before it turns into another unsuccessful night.

Action plan 2

1. In your diary write down the heading: My sleep environment. Now when you go to bed tonight, I want you to consciously think about the aforementioned topics, and make a note of the ones that apply to you:

Action	Yes/no
Do I feel safe in my environment?	
How can I feel even safer?	
Is my bedroom to bright at night?	
Should I use a sleep mask?	
Are my mattress and pillow as comfortable as possible?	

Is my sleepwear comfortable and breathable?	
Is there some kind of noise bothering me?	
Should I try using earplugs?	
What time you stopped looking at any form of LED lighting.	
Is my room is cool and ventilated?	
Have I removed my alarm or clock from arm's reach or keep it out of sight every morning?	
Does my environment smell pleasant?	
Has any of this helped me so far?	

Step 3: Get it together

3.1 Speak to your inner child

Try thinking of what used to help you fall asleep as a child. I don't mean you should give your mother a call and ask her to tell you a bedtime story, but if someone sang to you try listening to soft, relaxing music. If a parent used to read to you, try reading yourself. If you normally had a small snack such as a glass of milk before going to bed, try that too. Go back to what made you feel relaxed and safe, and try to replicate something similar. Rituals are put in place as an excellent way for children to feel safe and protected in their environment. As adults we often let the hustle and bustle of modern-day life tear us from our standard sleeping rituals, which could create feelings of stress and anxiety. It is important, even as an adult, to make sure your brain and body automatically know when it is time to sleep. Strong rituals will help you achieve this.

3.2 Start a schedule

Break your evening up into definite dedicated times. Firstly, get anything done that simply must be done before bedtime, such as washing the dishes or preparing lunch for the next day. These activities, when not complete, are often what keep us awake and anxious at night.

Thereafter, spend a small amount of time getting yourself ready for bed, and lastly, spend 20 minutes helping your body wind down with the helpful techniques discussed later in this book.

Try to wake up and go to bed at the same time each day. Keeping a 'before bed' ritual will slowly convince your brain that certain actions should lead to sleep. A simple example would be to have dinner at the same time each night, followed by a relaxing bath and reading a good book just before going to bed.
Try not to go to bed too early, even if you are completely drained. Try to stick to around the same time every night to get your internal clock to realise exactly when bedtime is.

Additionally, a good idea is to cut out sleeping in on weekends. Your brain supposedly likes routine, and disrupting this routine two out of seven days a week will inhibit your progress. If you simply cannot bear waking up early over the weekend, try extending it by only an hour, as opposed to lying in until midday. You can slowly lessen this length of time until you are able to comfortably wake up at the same time every day. If waking up is not your problem, do the reverse and slowly go to bed a little earlier each day until your week's sleep pattern is stable and consistent.

3.3 Cut down on quick Zs

Try not to nap in the afternoons. While people's opinions differ on whether napping promotes good sleep later at night or inhibits it, if you have only recently started napping in the afternoons, it could be that your brain already feels rested enough. This will ultimately throw out your sleep pattern and you may find you nap more in turn to catch up. By skipping napping you will be exhausting your energy fully before a proper bedtime. If you do feel the need to nap, try limiting it to no more than 30 minutes, and nowhere after 3pm.

3.4 Soak up

Take a warm bath before bed. Even better, throw in some soothing camomile or lavender bath salts. The warm water will relax your muscles and the fragrance will have a calming effect on your mind.

3.5 Don't force it

Don't go to bed when you're not tired, or especially if you start feeling anxious about not being able to fall asleep. If you are struggling to fall asleep, get up and do something relaxing like reading, or listen to some soft music until you are tired enough to go back to bed.

Avoid an afternoon slump. If you are consuming meals high in carbohydrates, chances are you are going to hit a major downer in the afternoon as your energy levels and blood-sugar levels drop. This will make you feel lethargic and in turn your body will burn less energy, leaving more energy when you're trying to fall asleep. This applies to snacks as well. If you are snacking on foods high in refined sugar in order to keep your energy levels up to get through the day, this can backfire in the same way as carbohydrates – with a massive decline in the afternoon. You want to keep your energy levels up and burn as much as possible during the day, so that your body is in dire need of refuelling when you need to sleep. If you do feel yourself becoming sluggish, take a step away from your desk and go for a short walk, or sit up straight and do a few deep-breathing techniques to get oxygen flowing through your body again.

Action plan 3

1. In your sleep diary, write down the heading "My sleep ritual". This is probably the most important page in your diary. You will more than likely revisit and redevelop this page as you learn more about your insomnia.

2. On this page, write down what your childhood ritual was like. Then write down how this has now changed.
3. Define your new sleep ritual dedicated times

Write down your dedicated bed time and wake up time

What was my childhood ritual like? Go into detail

How has this ritual now changed?

My Sleep ritual dedicated bed time:	
Time	How am I going to stay committed to this bed time?

My Sleep ritual dedicated wake up time:	
Time	What am I going to do to motivate myself to wake up now?

Step 4: Watch your mouth

4.1 Lose the stimulants

Limit caffeine and stimulants containing nicotine or sugar from the afternoon and especially before bedtime. They are called stimulants for a reason: they keep your brain awake and active, and could make it more difficult for you to fall asleep. You should try cutting out caffeine right from midday to see any real results, as it has a very long half-life and can remain in your system for many hours after consumption. Additionally, coffee is diuretic, which means it makes you urinate a lot, and this will lead to you waking up during the night. Something I figured out the hard way was that snacking on fruit in the afternoon was enough sugar to make it difficult for me to fall asleep.

Limit your alcohol intake before going to bed. While alcohol may initially help you to fall asleep, it could in fact inhibit the natural chemicals your brain releases to stay asleep. According to a study, this may be more prevalent in women. It may make you wake up more often during the night, interrupting your body's natural sleep cycle. It is essential to reach the deep stages of sleep to feel well rested in the morning. The same also applies to alcohol as coffee, in that both are diuretic.

4.2. Try cherry juice

Cherries are naturally high in melatonin, the natural sleep hormone your body releases to send you into a peaceful slumber. Studies showed that participants who drank pure cherry juice daily fell asleep sooner.

4.3 It's all about the size

Avoid large suppers at least two hours before going to sleep. When you eat heavy, rich foods, your stomach takes far longer to digest it. Additionally, spicy and acidic foods could cause heartburn and acid reflux. As mentioned earlier, this is one of the medical reasons you could be struggling with to fall asleep.

4.4 Warm milk

It seems your grandmother could have been onto something with this one. Some specialists believe it is due to a specific chemical found in milk called tryptophan, which helps your mind drift off into a peaceful slumber by assisting in the production of your body's natural serotonin (Serotonin plays an important role in the sleep cycle). Something interesting to note is that according to some scientists, if you are suffering from depression, it could be a sign that you potentially have a deficiency in tryptophan.

4.5 Check your meds

Make sure your prescriptions are not what's keeping you awake. There are many prescription drugs that list sleep disorders as a side effect. This could be anything from antidepressants to anti-inflammatory drugs. Check the label of your medication, or ask your local pharmacist if you think it could be the cause of your insomnia.

Melatonin is a natural hormone your body releases when your brain registers it is bedtime. You can also buy melatonin pills from a pharmacy to assist with sleep disruptions, but this has been known to cause fatigue the following day.

While sleeping pills can perhaps help to alleviate severe insomnia for a while, they are unlikely to help in the long term if there is an underlying psychological issue that needs to be addressed. Sleeping aids could even make it harder to fall asleep once you go off them.

Action plan 4

1. Make a quick note of what you eat each day and around what time. i.e 'apple and coffee, late afternoon'.
2. Double check any medication you have been using for possible stimulants or chemicals keeping you awake.

Breakfast

Snacks

Lunch

Snacks

Dinner

Any medication:

Step 5: Let's get physical

Being overweight is also linked to sleeping problems. Studies have shown that people who are more active are more likely to get a good night's sleep. Research has also shown that appetite-regulating hormones are directly affected by how well you sleep, and thus insomnia could actually lead to an increase in your weight by indirectly making you hungrier.

A study was conducted at Northwestern University that monitored middle-aged women in two groups. The first group was subjected to regular light aerobic activities, while the others had hobbies such as cooking classes. After a few months the study already showed that the ladies who were exercising regularly had improved sleep quality and quantity.

5.1 Exhaust your energy

Exercise is a fantastic way of not only relieving stress, but also exhausting all excess energy you may have. A good 30 minutes of cardio such as walking or cycling could help you feel more tired before bed, and in more need of a good night's sleep. Some professionals suggest not exercising from around four hours before bed, as you often feel wide awake and well energised just after physical activity. Most professionals will suggest exercising in the morning to not only get your blood flowing for the day, but also drain as much energy as possible while you are awake. This should allow you to wind down easily at night.

Personally, I really enjoy working out after work, as it clears my mind and really gets the oxygen flowing. I joined an exercise regimen for three months during which I woke up at 5am every morning, and exercised for an hour before work. I noticed a definite decrease in my energy levels before bedtime, and started going to bed much earlier to compensate for the lack of energy. So in my case this was a definite factor in fighting my insomnia. However, the reason why I say I still enjoy exercising after work is that in my opinion you are so tired after a full day's work and exercising in the morning that you end up having no social life at all. This was and is a large part of my life; I'm young and being around people makes me happy. So I had to find a way to make both work. This just goes to show that whatever suits your current situation, exercise is a very important part of any balanced lifestyle.

Another benefit of working out in the morning is that if you are bound to an exercise regimen, it is less likely for you to hit the snooze button and carry on sleeping. I found that if you have a definite time you have to wake up, especially if it is earlier than usual, your body gets into the habit of trying to get as much sleep as possible while it can. Hence you may fall asleep much more easily (you will just be a grumpy morning person if you are anything like me).

5.2 Salutation to the sun

Stretching exercises such as yoga can also assist in relieving bodily stress and strain, making it easier for you to fall asleep. You could even include five minutes of concentrated stretching into your bedtime ritual to make sure your body is completely relaxed and ready for sleep. I don't mean you need to whip out your yoga mat and pick the hardest pose; simply start stretching smaller, more concentrated parts of your body. You could start with easy head and shoulder rolls to loosen and stretch your neck and shoulders. Move down your body until all areas have been well stretched and you are feeling supple and relaxed.

5.3 #Lovethegym

Make exercise fun so that you don't even realise you are exercising. Do activities you enjoy, such as going for walks, playing with the dog or dancing. Exercising doesn't have to be tedious and boring by any means. And any exercise is always better than no exercise. A good guide would be the point at which your heart rate increases, or you begin breathing a lot deeper, while still being able to hold a conversation.

Action plan 5

1. Write down a dedicated time you are going to exercise each day
2. Write down all exercises you enjoy, such as walking or playing with the dog.

3. You may want to draw up a weekly roster you could stick to. You can change your activity for each week and keep it interesting and enjoyable.

Write down a dedicated time you are going to exercise each day
What exercises do I really enjoy?

Day	Activity
Monday	
Tuesday	
Wednesday	
Thursday	
Friday	
Saturday	
Sunday	

Step 6: Get rid of stress

6.1 Keep it outside the bedroom

Make sure that you don't do anything stressful in the bedroom. This could be anything from working on your laptop to arguing with your partner. The bedroom should be kept as a haven of relaxation and rest. Your mind should associate the bedroom only with going to sleep. I used to work on projects on my laptop while sitting on my bed, not thinking it would make any difference. Instead, what I found was that over the following days whenever I went to sleep, I would think about how I could improve on these projects instead of letting my brain shut down. I had begun associating the space with work as opposed to rest.

6.2 What's on your mind?

Keep a worry journal, or use a line in your sleep log to monitor this. This can help by allowing you an outlet from issues flooding your mind while you should be sleeping. Before going to bed, write down anything on your mind. This does not necessarily have to cause you stress, but could be anything that keeps your mind occupied. Once written down, promise yourself you are not going to allow yourself to be plagued by these worries until tomorrow morning. You will not forget them as you have written them down, and will be able to deal with them when you feel fresh and revived. A good suggestion is to speak with someone about your stresses, whether a professional or a close family member or friend. The act of getting it off your chest and knowing someone is there to listen to you will help you feel a little bit more secure and supported.

6.3 Smile

Get a more positive outlook on things that are worrying you. If this is the root cause, then it really is necessary that you delve deeper into what is stressing you out, and either start to change your situation or change your mindset about your situation. Try to minimise the negative thoughts you have around your daily life as well as your insomnia. As mentioned earlier, a good example to start with could be instead of saying, "I never sleep well at night, this is so frustrating," tell yourself, "There are many people who sometimes can't get a good night's rest. I am not the only one, this is not permanent and if I practise I will be able to sleep better." It takes time and practice to implement positive thinking permanently, but studies have shown that people with a more positive outlook tend to sleep better.

Action plan 6

1. If your work space is in the bedroom, move it to another room.
2. To improve your positivity, the first 2 things I want you to do when waking up

in the morning is to smile as big and bright as you can, and in your sleep journal I want you to write down 3 things you are grateful for. This can be anything, from being thankful for a wonderful family, to a good cup of hot coffee. You will immediately start your day with the right mindset.

3. In your sleep journal, name a page "Don't worry, be happy". Every night you feel you cannot sleep because you are worrying about something, write it down in a few sentences on this page, and then leave it there till you can sort it out the next day.

4. Any stresses you have sorted out you must then cross off your worry page with the biggest smile you can muster!

Day	3 things I am grateful for
Monday	
Tuesday	
Wednesday	
Thursday	
Friday	
Saturday	
Sunday	

Don't worry, be happy!

What is worrying me?	How did I sort this out?	Sorted!

Step 7: The ultimate chill-out guide

7.1 Chill out to some tunes

Listen to music or soothing sounds before going to bed. A lot of people find it comforting to fall asleep to soft music. The calmness and repetitive sound tends to help distract you from worrying thoughts and focus your mind on the serenity of falling asleep. I've also tried downloading a few sound-maker apps that play different soothing sounds to help me fall asleep.

7.2 Make it romantic

Many people use aromatherapy oils, specifically lavender, to induce sleep. Some studies have also showed that slight unpleasant smells when falling asleep can be linked to sleep disorders such as night terrors. Try spraying your pillow lightly with lavender or peppermint room spray.

7.3 Go for a massage

While we would all love regular massages to relieve stress and promote clear and focused thinking, a lot of us don't have the cash for a weekly professional massage. A great alternative is to ask your partner to help you with a short home-grown massage of even just 10 minutes. It doesn't necessarily matter that they are not professional, the light relaxing movements against your muscles as well as the loving physical contact should give you a feeling of relaxation and support.

7.4 Rock 'n roll

Okay, I'm not telling you to crank up some old-school rock tunes, but interestingly enough a group of Swiss researchers discovered that just as babies tend to fall asleep when being rocked in their parents' arms, the same applies for adults. Try buying yourself an old-school rocking chair to not only add some antique style to any lounge, but also coerce yourself into an infant-like state of sleep. While it may not entice you into falling asleep immediately, the slow rocking may allow you to fall asleep faster as well as enter a deep sleep state sooner.

7.5 Try mantram

Basically what you do is repeat a relaxing sentence, phrase or word in your mind over and over – almost like counting sheep or trying to hypnotise yourself. The repetitive effect is supposed to slowly relax your mind and keep out negative thoughts by keeping you lightly focused. This is helpful for people whose minds start to wonder with worry when they lie in bed.

7.6 Meditation for beginners

A simple meditation technique that focuses your mind on letting your body fall asleep is focused muscle relaxation. Basically what you do is slowly go through each of your body parts and make sure they are relaxed one by one. So when you are ready for bed and turn off the light, get into a comfortable position and start at your toes. Think about your toes and make sure all are relaxed; once this is so, move up your feet to your ankles, then lower legs, repeating the relaxation technique. Once you reach your head, concentrate on what sounds you can hear inside the room. Is there a soft fan on? Perhaps you can even hear your own breathing. Listen and explore all the soft night sounds you can hear within your room, and then shift your focus to outside your room. Is there a cricket outside your window? Perhaps it's raining or you can hear a few cars making their way home in the distance. Thereafter, use the relaxation technique once more, this time starting at the top of your head, going down all the way to your toes.

7.7 Take deep breaths

There are various breathing techniques that can also help to relax you before a good night's sleep. One I've tried is the following: Lie comfortably on your back and breathe in slowly and deeply through your nose for a count of five seconds. Hold your breath for 20 seconds, and then release through your mouth for 10 seconds, concentrating firstly on releasing the air from your stomach area and then through your chest. This exhale is similar to that of a baby, and we all know how most babies sleep.

Another simple technique used to slowly train yourself to take control of your own thoughts and focus is to allow and then decline yourself moments of conscious and precise thought in short intervals. For instance, keep a soft alarm next to your bed and time intervals of one minute. In the first minute, think and focus on one positive thought, such as how grateful you are for the lovely weather. Keep concentrating on this thought until the alarm rings. Now for the next minute, softly concentrate on only your breathing. Feel how air rushes in through your nose and fills your chest. Feel and concentrate on how your heart is beating, and then slowly release. On the next alarm, think once again of another positive thought, and repeat the process. As a beginner, aim for just a few minutes before bed, perhaps six minutes, and slowly move it up to 20 minutes.

You may find it difficult in the beginning to keep thoughts out of your head while you practise your breathing, but in this case practice makes perfect, and being able to focus and relax will in the long run become an essential skill at helping you fall asleep easily. Softly push the thought out of your mind and return to thinking of your breathing. Nothing should be negative or worrisome in this exercise.

7.8 The countdown begins

This was probably devised for the left-brain thinkers among us. Create a simple mathematical task for yourself where you count down from 100, skipping every third number, or count up to 200 in multiples of four. While mentally challenging, this technique is useful in keeping your mind distracted from anxious or negative thoughts before sleep. Don't be stressed about being 100% mathematically correct, just keep in mind the point of the task.

7.9 Lose control

This technique requires practice, but definitely helped me. You essentially concentrate on not concentrating at all. As complicated as this sounds, the reality of it is quite simple. When we go to bed we often have created thoughts, conversations and sentences we consciously run through our minds. The trick is to rather leave these types of thoughts at the door, and merely let your mind run whatever pictures it chooses. Think of it like going to a movie theatre, where you are not in control of the story at all, but someone else is showing you a stream of pictures.

Action plan 7

1. Create yourself a super sleep soundtrack
2. Make your sleep environment smell like a fresh spring field

3. Subtly hint to your partner just how helpful a soothing massage would be. You could even bribe them with delicious home baked goods.
4. See if you can't find or borrow a beautiful rocking chair to test drive
5. Try each of the following techniques over the next few evenings, using only one an evening. Then mark down on a scale of 1 to 10 how well each one worked for you. You could then concentrate on practicing the ones that worked best.
    a. Night 1: Mantram
    b. Night 2: Meditation
    c. Night 3: Deep breathing
    d. Night 4: Focused thoughts
    e. Night 5: The countdown
    f. Night 6: Lose control

Top 5 sleep soundtrack

Night	Activity	Did it help?
Night 1	Mantram	
Night 2	Meditation	
Night 3	Deep Breathing	

Night 4	Focused thoughts	
Night 5	The countdown	
Night 6	Lose control	

Step 8: Cognitive Behavioural Therapy (CBT) techniques

CBT is used specifically for breaking the cycle of insomnia and is helpful in changing thoughts and behaviour associated with anxiety before sleep. Because this attempts to treat the underlying problems associated with insomnia, it may have much longer lasting effects. This is normally performed by a clinical psychologist or GP, but there are also a number of simple techniques you could try to incorporate at home.

8.1 Sleep-restriction therapy

This is pretty self-explanatory. You intentionally limit your time in bed to the number of hours you actually sleep. In my case this was four hours. This may be frustrating at first, but the logic is that you'll spend less time awake in bed and can slowly increase the amount of sleep you get.

8.2 Paradoxical intention

This is a really fancy term for the concept of trying not to think about a pink elephant when someone tells you not to think about a pink elephant – and all of a sudden all you can think about is a pink elephant. So by telling yourself constantly not to fall asleep, you could trick your mind into actually falling asleep.

8.3 Biofeedback

A specialist in a monitored environment normally performs this, but you could quite simply apply the basic principle at home. The idea is just to monitor what makes you tense or uncomfortable and what makes you relax. If for instance you enjoy reading as part of your sleep ritual, but horror novels make you feel tense and alert, you may want to switch to soppy romance novels before bed.

Action plan 8

1. Try each of the following techniques over the next few evenings, using only one an evening. Mark down on a scale of 1 to 10 how well each worked for you. You could then concentrate on practicing the ones that worked best. Don't overlap these with the previous techniques until you have singled out exactly what is working best for you at the end of this book.
   a. Night 7: Sleep restriction therapy
   b. Night 8: Paradoxical intention
2. If you feel anxious or any negative feelings at all during the night or leading up to going to bed, write them down in your sleep journal.

Home CBT techniques

Technique	Did this help?
Sleep restriction therapy	
Paradoxical intention	

Step 9: Staying asleep

So you've somehow thankfully managed to fall asleep and now in the middle of your midnight miracle, you wake up for one reason or another. Perhaps a noise has woken you or you've had to quickly run to the bathroom. Whatever the case may be, you start stressing at the thought of all the work you've put into falling asleep and how you now have to do it all over again.

But there is no need to fret! You are already halfway there, and I find the techniques to staying asleep are in fact much easier than initially falling asleep.

9.1 Keep your focus

Firstly, stay calm and relaxed as you are and focus on your body's natural tiredness. Focus on how sleepy your head feels, how comfortable and cosy you are under your duvet, and what a lovely dream you were having.

9.2 Focus some more

Don't stress about falling asleep again, but rather just ultimate relaxation. Either way your body is in a wonderful state of rest, which will still help you to feel fresher.

9.3 Unwind again

If you really find that you are still just getting frustrated at the fact that you cannot fall back asleep, get out of bed and do a non-stimulating activity such as reading a book. Try to keep the lights turned down low so as not to reawaken yourself.

Action plan 9

1. Stay focused and keep calming yourself using your affirmations or the simple techniques you found worked best for you.

When to seek professional help

If after trying all of the above techniques for a manageable period of time, you still find you are struggling to fall asleep or are at least not improving, you may need to seek professional help from your GP. They may refer you to a psychologist, who will assist in treating any underlying psychological stress you could be suffering from. Psychological stress can range from mood disorders such as depression to anxiety and psychotic disorders.

Alternatively, you could also be suffering from underlying physical health disorders such as heart and respiratory problems, hormonal issues or chronic pain.

This list of techniques and your sleep diary can be used to assist you in properly explaining to your healthcare professional what you have already tried and could possibly eliminate as a cause.

Conclusion

Congratulations on taking the first step to achieving serene and peaceful sleep. I truly hope the sleep log we created as well as the techniques in this book helped you to gain a better understanding of why you're not sleeping, and possibly helped you develop your own sleep ritual to switch off your brain, sleep better and feel refreshed!

I would love to know any comments you have on my book, what helped you, what didn't help you, or what you would love to know more about. I would really appreciate your review in order to make this guide even better for future readers also battling to sleep!

We would love if you would leave a review! Thank you for taking the time to help us out.

The mellowzoo team

http://www.mellowzoo.com

Please scroll down for some sneak previews to books we think will further help you!

About the author

Dene Chittenden wrote her first ebook at the age of 27 after realizing insomnia offers you a lot of time you never had before, to do things like write books about how horrible it is to suffer from insomnia. Since then her sleeping habits have improved but alas her love for small yappy dogs has not. After earning her Honours in Information Design from the University of Pretoria she worked as a graphic designer for a local publishing company, and then as a design specialist and marketing assistant for a global corporation.

A die-hard traveller at heart, Dene will always be a born and bred, home-grown South African with a built in need for a thick steak and sunny skies. She currently lives in the capital city of Pretoria with her husband, and when she's not busy writing her next easy-to-follow self-help ebook you can find her cruising the streets for the latest hot foodie spot, flying to Cape Town for a local wine fest or indulging in her unhealthy addiction to local music.

She is releasing a blog in the near future focusing on self help topics aimed at an audience with a busy mind and not much time. Sign up for the free audiobook and we will notify you as soon as it is up and running, as well as any exclusive specials we may have for our subscribers.

PREVIEW OF: "TIME MANAGEMENT: 12 SIMPLE TIME MANAGEMENT STEPS TO BETTER FOCUS, FASTER PROGRESS AND OPTIMAL RESULTS"

"Productivity is not just about doing more, it is about creating more impact with less work."
– Prima Malik

Time is a finite commodity; we have only the allotted number of hours in a day to get things done. And if you're anything like the millions of people out there trying to keep up in this always-on, always-connected digital age, it might seem like those hours just aren't enough.

But what if you changed the way you used those hours? The simple fact is that successful people manage their time better. It's not about trying to do more, it's about streamlining what you're already doing – focusing enough time on the right tasks – and in that way opening up more time for other pursuits, like those things you've always wanted to do, but can never get around to.

That's the topic this book explores: harnessing good time management, sharper focus and correct planning to make every 24 hours as productive as they can possibly be. It's really that easy. You just need to change your approach.

So if you're ready to super-charge what you're really capable of accomplishing every day, let's get started!

Search time management by Joshua Nathan on the Amazon Kindle Store

---

"Most humans are never fully present in the now, because unconsciously they believe that the next moment must be more important than this one. But then you miss your whole life, which is never not now. And that's a revelation for some people: to realise that your life is only ever now." – Eckhart Tolle

---

Have you ever walked into a room and forgotten why you went there in the first place? Have you ever driven somewhere with absolutely no memory of how you got there? Do you often knock things over or bump into things?
That's because you're functioning *mindlessly*, instead of *mindfully*. Your brain is on auto-pilot – its default mode network (DMN). This is the area of the brain that kicks into action when you're not focused on the outside world; when your mind is wandering or daydreaming (known colloquially as "monkey mind"). It's a state of being that makes you miss out on life.

We have become so inclined to be mindless, as our minds seek refuge from the extreme stress and repetitive monotony of everyday life. We love to obsess over things that happened yesterday and things that are still to come.

And our days are consumed by work – the busier we are, the less we notice time passing by. Then we get home, plop down on the couch, and spend the rest of the day staring at the TV or pursuing another mindless activity. It's something many look forward to as an escape; an opportunity to just shut down. But that's an entire day of which we'll remember little the next day, and nothing a week later. That's a day, a week, a year you spent focused on everything *but* the present moment, and missed beautiful life happening all around you.

Think about how much time you spend walking around on auto-pilot, only ever paying attention when someone says your name. What's happening around you right now – the sounds, the smells, the atmosphere. Have you noticed any of it?

It's time to become **mindful** – noticing, experiencing and appreciating the present more; learning to savour the moment and create more memorable ones; reinforcing bonds with the people in your life by paying attention to them; taking care of your body and mind the way they deserve; and easing the stress of everyday living by increasing your understanding of yourself. This book is an aid to help you snap out of it for good, and actually live in the moment. After all, the only time that really exists is the present. It's all you have, and all you ever will have. You cannot change the past; and the future is forever out of reach. Life is such a precious gift – stop letting it pass you by.

Try these 12 simple steps, and I guarantee you'll walk out of the experience with a new perspective – and hopefully as a happier, less stressed and more present human being, who'll live a fuller life as a consequence.
So are you ready to live in the moment? Let's get started!

Search Mindfulness by Joshua Nathan on the Amazon Kindle Store

www.ingramcontent.com/pod-product-compliance
Lightning Source LLC
Chambersburg PA
CBHW071243280526
45788CB00004B/1563